My Ketogenic Air Fryer Lunch

A Set of Mouth-Watering Recipes for Delicious Ketogenic Air Fryer Meals

Michael Clark

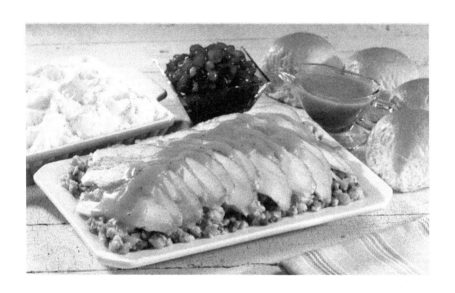

advice. The content within this book has been derived from various sources. Please consult a licensed professional before attempting any techniques outlined in this book.

By reading this document, the reader agrees that under no circumstances is the author responsible for any losses, direct or indirect, which are incurred as a result of the use of information contained within this document, including, but not limited to, — errors, omissions, or inaccuracies.

Table of Contents

Spiced Beef Meatballs

Prep time: 15 minutes

Cooking time: 10 minutes

Servings: 2

Ingredients:

- 1 oz pimiento jalapenos, pickled, chopped
- ½ teaspoon dried rosemary
- ½ teaspoon salt
- 9 oz ground beef
- ½ teaspoon ground coriander
- ¼ teaspoon ground nutmeg
- 1 egg, beaten
- 2 oz provolone cheese, shredded
- 2 teaspoons mascarpone
- ¼ teaspoon minced garlic
- Cooking spray

Directions:

1. In the mixing bowl mix up pickled pimiento jalapenos, dried rosemary, salt, ground beef, coriander, nutmeg, egg, and make the medium-size meatballs. Preheat the air fryer to 365F. Then spray the air fryer basket with cooking spray and place the meatballs inside. Cook the meatballs for 6 minutes, Then carefully flip them on another side and cook for 4 minutes more. Meanwhile, churn together minced garlic and mascarpone. When the meatballs are cooked, transfer them in the serving plates and top with garlic mascarpone.

Nutrition: calories 385, fat 18.5, fiber 0.7, carbs 2.3, protein 49.4

Chili Bell Peppers Stew

Preparation time: 5 minutes

Cooking time: 15 minutes

Servings: 4

Ingredients:

- red bell peppers, cut into wedges
- 2 green bell peppers, cut into wedges 2 yellow bell peppers, cut into wedges
- ½ cup keto tomato sauce 1 tablespoon chili powder
- 2 teaspoons cumin, ground
- ¼ teaspoon sweet paprika
- Salt and black pepper to the taste

Directions:

1. In a pan that fits your air fryer, mix all the ingredients, toss, introduce the pan in the machine and cook at 370 degrees F for 15 minutes. Divide into bowls and serve for lunch.

Nutrition: calories 190, fat 4, fiber 2, carbs 4, protein 7

Bacon Pancetta Casserole

Prep time: 10 minutes

Cooking time: 20 minutes

Servings: 4

Ingredients:

- 2 cups cauliflower, shredded

- 3 oz pancetta, chopped

- 2 oz bacon, chopped

- 1 cup Cheddar cheese, shredded

- ½ cup heavy cream

- 1 teaspoon salt

- 1 teaspoon cayenne pepper

- 1 teaspoon dried oregano

Directions:

1.   Put bacon and pancetta in the air fryer and cook it for 10 minutes at 400F. Stir the ingredients every 3 minutes to avoid burning. Then mix up shredded cauliflower and cooked pancetta and bacon. Add salt and

14

cayenne pepper. Mix up the mixture. Add the dried oregano. Line the air fryer pan with baking paper and put the cauliflower mixture inside. Top it with Cheddar cheese and sprinkle with heavy cream. Cook the casserole for 10 minutes at 365F.

Nutrition: calories 381, fat 30.5, fiber 1.5, carbs 4.5, protein 22.1

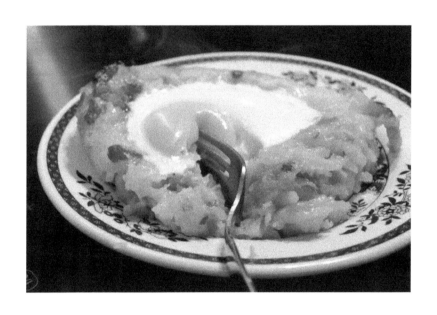

Okra and Peppers Casserole

Preparation time: 5 minutes

Cooking time: 20 minutes

Servings: 4

Ingredients:

- teaspoon olive oil 3 cups okra

- red bell peppers, cubed

- Salt and black pepper to the taste 2 tomatoes, chopped

- garlic cloves, minced

- ¼ cup keto tomato sauce

- 2 teaspoons coriander, ground 1 tablespoon cilantro, chopped

- ½ cup cheddar, shredded

Directions:

1.   Grease a heat proof dish that fits your air fryer with the oil, add all the ingredients except the cilantro and the cheese and toss them really gently. Sprinkle the cheese

17

and the cilantro on top, introduce the dish in the fryer and cook at 390 degrees F for 20 minutes. Divide between plates and serve for lunch.

Nutrition: calories 221, fat 7, fiber 2, carbs 4, protein 9

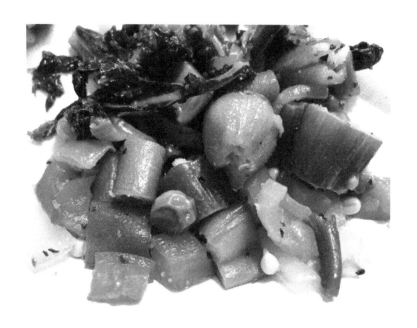

Cheese Pies

Prep time: 15 minutes

Cooking time: 4 minutes

Servings: 4

Ingredients:

- 8 wonton wraps

- 1 egg, beaten

- 1 cup cottage cheese

- 1 tablespoon Erythritol

- ½ teaspoon vanilla extract

- 1 egg white, whisked

- Cooking spray

Directions:

1. Mix up cottage cheese and Erythritol. Then add vanilla extract and egg. Stir the mixture well with the help of the fork. After this, put the cottage cheese mixture on the wonton wraps and fold them in the shape of pies. Then brush the pies with whisked egg white.

Preheat the air fryer to 375F. Then put the cottage cheese pies in the air fryer and spray them with the cooking spray. Cook the meal for 2 minutes from each side.

Nutrition: calories 92, fat 2.2, fiber 0, carbs 6.3, protein 11

Tomato Casserole

Preparation time: 5 minutes

Cooking time: 20 minutes

Servings: 4

Ingredients:

- tablespoon olive oil

- spring onions, chopped 3 garlic cloves, minced

- 1 teaspoon smoked paprika 1 tablespoon thyme, dried 2 celery sticks, sliced

- 1 yellow bell pepper, chopped

- 14 ounces cherry tomatoes, cubed 2 courgettes, sliced

- ½ cup mozzarella, shredded

Directions:

1. In a baking dish that fits your air fryer, mix all the ingredients except the cheese and toss. Sprinkle the cheese on top, introduce the dish in your air fryer and

cook at 380 degrees F for 20 minutes. Divide between plates and serve for lunch.

Nutrition: calories 254, fat 12, fiber 2, carbs 4, protein 11

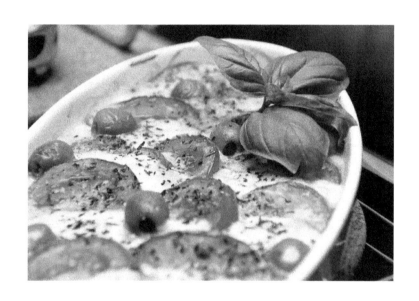

Chicken Stuffed Eggplants

Prep time: 20 minutes

Cooking time: 20 minutes

Servings: 4

Ingredients:

- 1-pound mini eggplants
- 1 tomato, chopped
- 2 oz Feta cheese, crumbled
- 1 teaspoon fresh parsley, chopped
- ¼ teaspoon salt
- 9 oz ground chicken
- ½ teaspoon fennel seeds
- 1 teaspoon minced garlic
- 1 tablespoon ghee
- 1 teaspoon salt
- 1 cup of water
- Cooking spray

Directions:

1.   Make the pockets in the eggplants by removing eggplant meat from them. Then sprinkle the eggplants with 1 teaspoon of salt and put in the water for 10-15 minutes. After this, preheat the air fryer to 365F. Dry the eggplants and place them in the air fryer in one layer. Spray them with the cooking spray and cook for 10 minutes at 365F. Meanwhile, put ghee in the skillet and melt it over the medium heat. Add parsley, tomato, ¼ teaspoon of salt, ground chicken, and minced garlic. Add fennel seeds and cook the ingredients for 10 minutes over the medium heat. When the eggplants are cooked, remove them from the air fryer and cool to the room temperature. Fill the eggplants with ground chicken mixture.

Nutrition: calories 229, fat 11.3, fiber 3.2, carbs 10.8, protein 21.6

Smoked Chicken mix

Preparation time: 5 minutes

Cooking time: 25 minutes

Servings: 4

Ingredients:

- and ½ pound chicken breasts, skinless, boneless and cubed Salt and black pepper to the taste

- ½ cup chicken stock

- teaspoons smoked paprika

- ½ teaspoon basil, dried

Directions:

1. In a pan that fits the air fryer, combine all the ingredients, toss, introduce the pan in the fryer and cook at 390 degrees F for 25 minutes. Divide between plates and serve for lunch with a side salad.

Nutrition: calories 223, fat 12, fiber 2, carbs 5, protein 13

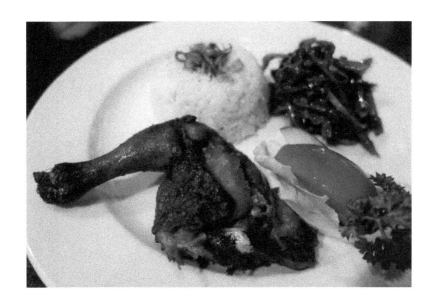

Almond Chicken Curry

Prep time: 10 minutes

Cooking time: 15 minutes

Servings: 2

Ingredients:

- 10 oz chicken fillet, chopped
- 1 teaspoon ground turmeric
- ½ cup spring onions, diced
- 1 teaspoon salt
- ½ teaspoon curry powder
- ½ teaspoon garlic, diced
- ½ teaspoon ground coriander
- ½ cup of organic almond milk
- 1 teaspoon Truvia
- 1 teaspoon olive oil

Directions:

1.   Put the chicken in the bowl. Add the ground turmeric, salt, curry powder, diced garlic, ground coriander, and almond Truvia. Then add olive oil and mix up the chicken. After this, add almond milk and transfer the chicken in the air fryer pan. Then preheat the air fryer to 375F and place the pan with korma curry inside. Top the chicken with diced onion. Cook the meal for 10 minutes. Stir it after 5 minutes of cooking. If the chicken is not cooked after 10 minutes, cook it for an additional 5 minutes.

Nutrition: calories 327, fat 14.5, fiber 1.5, carbs 5.6, protein 42

Cabbage Stew

Preparation time: 5 minutes

Cooking time: 20 minutes

Servings: 4

Ingredients:

- 14 ounces tomatoes, chopped

- 1 green cabbage head, shredded Salt and black pepper to the taste 1 tablespoon sweet paprika

- 4 ounces chicken stock

- 2 tablespoon dill, chopped

Directions:

1.   In a pan that fits your air fryer, mix the cabbage with the tomatoes and all the other ingredients except the dill, toss, introduce the pan in the fryer, and cook at 380 degrees F for 20 minutes. Divide into bowls and serve with dill sprinkled on top.

Nutrition: calories 200, fat 8, fiber 3, carbs 4, protein 6

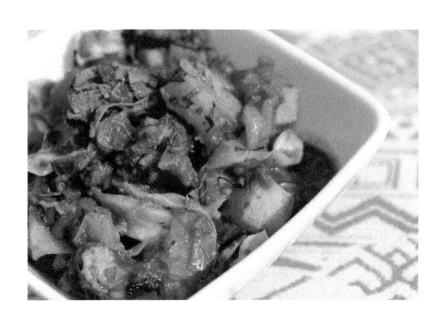

Mozzarella Cups

Prep time: 10 minutes

Cooking time: 6 minutes

Servings: 2

Ingredients:

- 2 eggs
- 2 oz Mozzarella, grated
- 1 oz Parmesan, grated
- 1 teaspoon coconut oil, melted
- ¼ teaspoon chili powder

Directions:

1.   Crack the eggs and separate egg yolks and egg whites. Then whisk the egg whites till the soft peaks. Separately whisk the egg yolks until smooth and add chili powder. Then carefully add egg whites, Parmesan, and Mozzarella. Stir the ingredients. Brush the silicone egg molds with coconut oil. Then put the cheese-egg mixture in the molds with the help of the spoon. Transfer the molds in the air fryer and cook at 385F for 6 minutes.

Nutrition: calories 209, fat 14.7, fiber 0.1, carbs 2, protein 18.1

Coconut Pudding

Preparation time: 5 minutes

Cooking time: 20 minutes

Servings: 4

Ingredients:

- cup cauliflower rice
- ½ cup coconut, shredded 3 cups coconut milk
- tablespoons stevia

Directions:

1.   In a pan that fits the air fryer, combine all the ingredients and whisk well. Introduce the in your air fryer and cook at 360 degrees F for 20 minutes. Divide into bowls and serve for breakfast.

Nutrition: calories 211, fat 11, fiber 3, carbs 4, protein 8

Cheesy Pancake

Prep time: 10 minutes

Cooking time: 8 minutes

Servings: 2

Ingredients:

- 5 eggs, beaten
- ¼ cup almond flour
- ½ teaspoon baking powder
- 1 teaspoon apple cider vinegar
- ¼ cup Cheddar cheese, shredded
- 1 teaspoon butter
- 1 tablespoon mascarpone
- ½ teaspoon sesame oil

Directions:

1. Brush the air fryer basket with sesame oil. Then in the mixing bowl mix up all remaining ingredients. Stir the liquid until homogenous. Pour it in the air fryer pan and place it in the air fryer. Cook the pancake for 8 minutes

at 360F. Remove the cooked pancake from the air fryer pan and cut it into servings.

Nutrition: calories 276, fat 21.4, fiber 0.4, carbs 2.6, protein 19

Mozzarella Bell Peppers Mix

Preparation time: 5 minutes

Cooking time: 15 minutes

Servings: 4

Ingredients:

• red bell pepper, roughly chopped 1 celery stalk, chopped

• green onions, sliced

• 2 tablespoons butter, melted

• ½ cup mozzarella cheese, shredded A pinch of salt and black pepper

• 6 eggs, whisked

Directions:

1. In a bowl, mix all the ingredients except the butter and whisk well. Preheat the air fryer at 360 degrees F, add the butter, heat it up, add the celery and bell peppers mix, and cook for 15 minutes, shaking the fryer once. Divide the mix between plates and serve for breakfast.

Nutrition: calories 222, fat 12, fiber 4, carbs 5, protein 7

Scallion Eggs Bake

Prep time: 10 minutes

Cooking time: 20 minutes

Servings: 2

Ingredients:

- 2 eggs
- 4 oz double Gloucester cheese, grated'
- 1 teaspoon coconut flour
- ¼ cup heavy cream
- 1 tablespoon butter
- 1 tablespoon scallions, chopped

Directions:

1.   Place the eggs on the rack and insert the rack in the air fryer. Cook the eggs for 17 minutes at 250F. Then cool the eggs in cold water and peel. Cut the eggs into halves. In the bowl mix up cheese, heavy cream, butter, and coconut flour. Microwave the mixture for 1 minute or until it is liquid. Place the egg halves in the 2 ramekins.

Pour the cheese mixture over the eggs and top with scallions. Place the ramekins in the air fryer and cook them for 3 minutes at 400F.

Nutrition: calories 395, fat 36.2, fiber 0.6, carbs 1.7, protein 20.4

Oregano and Coconut Scramble

Preparation time: 5 minutes

Cooking time: 20 minutes

Servings: 4

Ingredients:

- 8 eggs, whisked
- 2 tablespoons oregano, chopped Salt and black pepper to the taste 2 tablespoons parmesan, grated
- ¼ cup coconut cream

Directions:

1. In a bowl, mix the eggs with all the ingredients and whisk. Pour this into a pan that fits your air fryer, introduce it in the preheated fryer and cook at 350 degrees F for 20 minutes, stirring often. Divide the scramble between plates and serve for breakfast.

Nutrition: calories 221, fat 12, fiber 4, carbs 5, protein 9

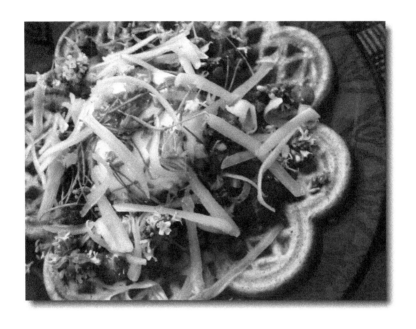

Chia and Hemp Pudding

Prep time: 4 hours

Cooking time: 2 minutes

Servings: 2

Ingredients:

- 1 teaspoon hemp seeds

- 1 teaspoon chia seeds

- 1 tablespoon almond flour

- 1 teaspoon coconut flakes

- 1 teaspoon walnuts, chopped

- ½ teaspoon flax meal

- ¼ teaspoon vanilla extract

- ½ teaspoon Erythritol

- ½ cup of coconut milk

- ¼ cup water, boiled

Directions:

1.   Put hemp seeds, chia seeds, almond flour, coconut flakes, walnuts, flax meal, vanilla extract, coconut milk, and water in the big bowl. Stir the mixture until homogenous and pour it into 2 mason jars. Leave the mason jars in the cold place for 4 hours. Then top the surface of the pudding with Erythritol. Place the mason jars in the air fryer and cook the pudding for 2 minutes at 400F or until you get the light brown crust.

Nutrition: calories 257, fat 24.2, fiber 4.4, carbs 8.4, protein 5.8

Zucchini Salad

Preparation time: 4 minutes

Cooking time: 15 minutes

Servings: 2

Ingredients:

- cup watercress, torn 1 tablespoon olive oil

- cups zucchini, roughly cubed 1 cup parmesan cheese, grated Cooking spray.

Directions:

1.   Grease a pan that fits the air fryer with the cooking spray, add all the ingredients except the cheese, sprinkle the cheese on top and cook at 390 degrees F for 15 minutes. Divide into bowls and serve for breakfast.

Nutrition: calories 202, fat 11, fiber 3, carbs 5, protein 4

Sausages Squares

Prep time: 20 minutes

Cooking time: 20 minutes

Servings: 4

Ingredients:

- ½ cup almond flour

- ¼ cup butter, melted

- 1 egg yolk

- ½ teaspoon baking powder

- ¼ teaspoon salt

- 6 oz sausage meat

- ¼ teaspoon ground black pepper

- Cooking spray

Directions:

1.   Make the dough: in the mixing bowl mix up almond flour, butter, egg yolk, and baking powder. Add salt and knead the non-sticky dough. In the separated bowl mix up ground black pepper and sausage meat. Roll up the

dough with the help of the rolling pin. Then cut the dough into squares.

2.   Place the sausage meat in the center of dough squares and secure them in the shape of the puff. Then preheat the air fryer to 320F. Line the air fryer basket with baking paper. Put the sausage puffs over the baking paper and spray them with cooking spray. Cook the meal for 20 minutes at 325F.

Nutrition: calories 280, fat 26.5, fiber 0.4, carbs 1.3, protein 9.8

Tomato and Greens Salad

Preparation time: 5 minutes

Cooking time: 15 minutes

Servings: 4

Ingredients:

- teaspoon olive oil

- cups mustard greens

- A pinch of salt and black pepper

- ½ pound cherry tomatoes, cubed 2 tablespoons chives, chopped

Directions:

1. Heat up your air fryer with the oil at 360 degrees F, add all the ingredients, toss, cook for 15 minutes shaking halfway, divide into bowls and serve for breakfast.

Nutrition: calories 224, fat 8, fiber 2, carbs 3, protein 7

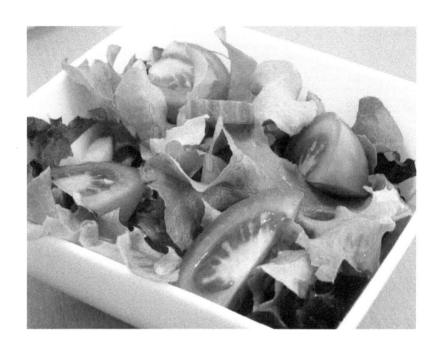

Turmeric Salmon and Cauliflower Rice

Preparation time: 5 minutes

Cooking time: 25 minutes

Servings: 4

Ingredients:

• 4 salmon fillets, boneless

• Salt and black pepper to the taste 1 cup cauliflower, riced

• ½ cup chicken stock

• 1 teaspoon turmeric powder 1 tablespoon butter, melted

Directions:

1. In a pan that fits your air fryer, mix the cauliflower rice with the other ingredients except the salmon and toss. Arrange the salmon fillets over the cauliflower rice, put the pan in the fryer and cook at 360 degrees F for 25 minutes, flipping the fish after 15 minutes. Divide everything between plates and serve.

Nutrition: calories 241, fat 12, fiber 2, carbs 6, protein 12

Oregano Salmon

Prep time: 10 minutes

Cooking time: 7 minutes

Servings: 2

Ingredients:

- 10 oz salmon fillet
- 1 teaspoon dried oregano
- 1 teaspoon sesame oil
- 2 oz Parmesan, grated
- ¼ teaspoon chili flakes

Directions:

1. Sprinkle the salmon fillet with dried oregano and chili flakes. Then brush it with sesame oil. Preheat the air fryer to 385F. Place the salmon in the air fryer basket and cook it for 5 minutes. Then flip the fish on another side and top with Parmesan. Cook the fish for 2 minutes more.

Nutrition: calories 301, fat 17.2, fiber 0.3, carbs 1.5, protein 36.7

Minty Trout and Pine Nuts

Preparation time: 5 minutes

Cooking time: 16 minutes

Servings: 4

Ingredients:

- 4 rainbow trout

- 1 cup olive oil + 3 tablespoons Juice of 1 lemon

- A pinch of salt and black pepper 1 cup parsley, chopped

- 3 garlic cloves, minced

- ½ cup mint, chopped Zest of 1 lemon

- 1/3 pine nuts

- 1 avocado, peeled, pitted and roughly chopped

Directions:

1.   Pat dry the trout, season with salt and pepper and rub with 3 tablespoons oil. Put the fish in your air fryer's basket and cook for 8 minutes on each side. Divide the fish between plates and drizzle half of the lemon juice all

over. In a blender, combine the rest of the oil with the remaining lemon juice, parsley, garlic, mint, lemon zest, pine nuts and the avocado and pulse well. Spread this over the trout and serve.

Nutrition: calories 240, fat 12, fiber 4, carbs 6, protein 9

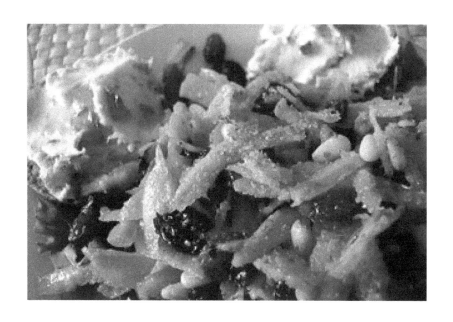

Fried Anchovies

Prep time: 20 minutes

Cooking time: 6 minutes

Servings: 4

Ingredients:

- 1-pound anchovies

- ¼ cup coconut flour

- 2 eggs, beaten

- 1 teaspoon salt

- 1 teaspoon ground black pepper

- 1 tablespoon lemon juice

- 1 tablespoon sesame oil

Directions:

1. Trim and wash anchovies if needed and put in the big bowl. Add salt and ground black pepper. Mix up the anchovies. Then add eggs and stir the fish until you get a homogenous mixture. After this coat every anchovies fish in the coconut flour. Brush the air fryer pan with

sesame oil. Place the anchovies in the pan in one layer. Preheat the air fryer to 400F. Put the pan with anchovies in the air fryer and cook them for 6 minutes or until anchovies are golden brown.

Nutrition: calories 332, fat 17.7, fiber 2.7, carbs 4.6, protein 36.6

Herbed Trout Mix

Preparation time: 5 minutes

Cooking time: 20 minutes

Servings: 4

Ingredients:

- 4 trout fillets, boneless and skinless 1 tablespoon lemon juice

- 2 tablespoons olive oil

- A pinch of salt and black pepper 1 bunch asparagus, trimmed

- 2 tablespoons ghee, melted

- ¼ cup mixed chives and tarragon

Directions:

1. Mix the asparagus with half of the oil, salt and pepper, put it in your air fryer's basket, cook at 380 degrees F for 6 minutes and divide between plates. In a bowl, mix the trout with salt, pepper, lemon juice, the rest of the oil and the herbes and toss, Put the fillets in your air fryer's basket and cook at 380 degrees F for 7

minutes on each side. Divide the fish next to the asparagus, drizzle the melted ghee all over and serve.

Nutrition: calories 240, fat 12, fiber 4, carbs 6, protein 9

Tilapia Bowls

Prep time: 15 minutes

Cooking time: 10 minutes

Servings: 4

Ingredients:

- 7 oz tilapia fillet or flathead fish

- 1 teaspoon arrowroot powder

- 1 teaspoon ground paprika

- ½ teaspoon salt

- ½ teaspoon ground black pepper

- ¼ teaspoon ground cumin

- ½ teaspoon garlic powder

- 1 teaspoon lemon juice

- 4 oz purple cabbage, shredded

- 1 jalapeno, sliced

- 1 tablespoon heavy cream

- ½ teaspoon minced garlic

- Cooking spray

Directions:

1.   Sprinkle the tilapia fillet with arrowroot powder, ground paprika, salt, ground black pepper, ground cumin, and garlic powder. Preheat the air fryer to 385F. Spray the tilapia fillet with cooking spray and place it in the air fryer. Cook the fish for 10 minutes. Meanwhile, in the bowl mix up shredded cabbage, jalapeno pepper, and lemon juice. When the tilapia fillet is cooked, chop it roughly. Put the shredded cabbage mixture in the serving bowls. Top them with chopped tilapia. After this, in the shallow bowl mix up minced garlic and heavy cream. Sprinkle the meal with a heavy cream mixture.

Nutrition: calories 69, fat 2, fiber 1.1, carbs 3.6, protein 9.9

Cilantro Salmon

Preparation time: 5 minutes

Cooking time: 12 minutes

Servings: 4

Ingredients:

- 4 salmon fillets, boneless Juice of ½ lemon
- ¼ cup chives, chopped
- 4 cilantro springs, chopped 3 tablespoons olive oil
- Salt and black pepper to the taste

Directions:

1.   In a bowl, mix the salmon with all the other ingredients and toss. Put the fillets in your air fryer's basket and cook at 370 degrees F for 12 minutes, flipping the fish halfway. Divide everything between plates and serve with a side salad.

Nutrition: calories 240, fat 12, fiber 5, carbs 6, protein 14

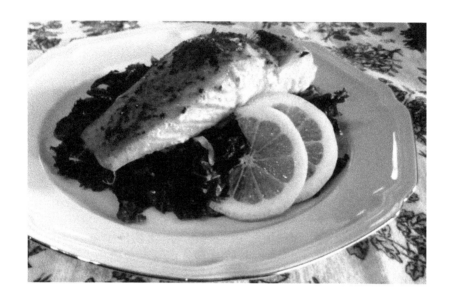

Mahi Mahi and Broccoli Cakes

Prep time: 15 minutes

Cooking time: 11 minutes

Servings: 4

Ingredients:

- ½ cup broccoli, shredded
- 1 tablespoon flax meal
- 1 egg, beaten
- 1 teaspoon ground coriander
- 1 oz Monterey Jack cheese, shredded
- ½ teaspoon salt
- 6 oz Mahi Mahi, chopped
- Cooking spray

Directions:

1.   In the mixing bowl mix up flax meal, egg, ground coriander, salt, broccoli, and chopped Mahi Mahi. Stir the ingredients gently with the help of the fork and add shredded Monterey Jack cheese. Stir the mixture until

homogenous. Then make 4 cakes. Preheat the air fryer to 390F. Place the Mahi Mahi cakes in the air fryer and spray them gently with cooking spray. Cook the fish cakes for 5 minutes and then flip on another side.

2.   Cook the fish cakes for 6 minutes more.

Nutrition: calories 90, fat 4.2, fiber 0.8, carbs 1.4, protein 11.7

Balsamic Trouts with Tomatoes and Pepper

Preparation time: 5 minutes

Cooking time: 16 minutes

Servings: 2

Ingredients:

- 2 trout fillets, boneless 2 tomatoes, cubed

- 1 red bell pepper, chopped 2 garlic cloves, minced

- 1 tablespoon olive oil

- tablespoon balsamic vinegar A pinch of salt and black pepper 2 tablespoon almond flakes

Directions:

1. Arrange the fish in a pan that fits your air fryer, add the rest of the ingredients and toss gently. Cook at 370 degrees F for 16 minutes, divide between plates and serve.

Nutrition: calories 261, fat 14, fiber 5, carbs 6, protein 14

Squid Stuffed with Cauliflower Mix

Prep time: 20 minutes

Cooking time: 6 minutes

Servings: 4

Ingredients:

• 4 squid tubes, trimmed

• 1 teaspoon ground paprika

• ½ teaspoon ground turmeric

• ½ teaspoon garlic, diced

• ½ cup cauliflower, shredded

• 1 egg, beaten

• ½ teaspoon salt

• ½ teaspoon ground ginger

• Cooking spray

Directions:

1. Clean the squid tubes if needed. After this, in the mixing bowl mix up ground paprika, turmeric, garlic,

shredded cauliflower, salt, and ground ginger. Stir the mixture gently and add a beaten egg. Mix the mixture up. Then fill the squid tubes with shredded cauliflower mixture. Secure the edges of the squid tubes with toothpicks. Preheat the air fryer to 390F. Place the stuffed squid tubes in the air fryer and spray with cooking spray. Cook the meal for 6 minutes.

Nutrition: calories 8., fat 2.7, fiber 0.6, carbs 1.5, protein 13.8

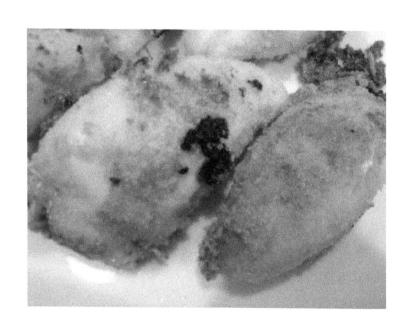

Chia Cinnamon Pudding

Preparation time: 10 minutes

Cooking time: 25 minutes

Servings: 6

Ingredients:

- cups coconut cream 6 egg yolks, whisked 2 tablespoons stevia

- ¼ cup chia seeds

- 2 teaspoons cinnamon powder 1 tablespoon ghee, melted

Directions:

1. In a bowl, mix all the ingredients, whisk, divide into 6 ramekins, place them all in your air fryer and cook at 340 degrees F for 25 minutes. Cool the puddings down and serve.

Nutrition: calories 180, fat 4, fiber 2 carbs 5, protein 7

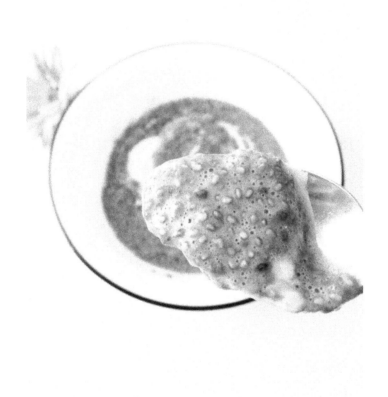

Seeds and Almond Cookies

Prep time: 15 minutes

Cooking time: 9 minutes

Servings: 6

Ingredients:

- 1 teaspoon chia seeds

- 1 teaspoon sesame seeds

- 1 tablespoon pumpkin seeds, crushed

- 1 egg, beaten

- 2 tablespoons Splenda

- 1 teaspoon vanilla extract

- 1 tablespoon butter

- 4 tablespoons almond flour

- ¼ teaspoon ground cloves

- 1 teaspoon avocado oil

Directions:

1. Put the chia seeds, sesame seeds, and pumpkin seeds in the bowl. Add egg, Splenda, vanilla extract, butter, avocado oil, and ground cloves. Then add almond flour and mix up the mixture until homogenous. Preheat the air fryer to 375F. Line the air fryer basket with baking paper. With the help of the scooper make the cookies and flatten them gently. Place the cookies in the air fryer. Arrange them in one layer. Cook the seeds cookies for 9 minutes.

Nutrition: calories 180, fat 13.7, fiber 3, carbs 9.6, protein 5.8

Cauliflower Rice Pudding

Preparation time: 5 minutes

Cooking time: 25 minutes

Servings: 4

Ingredients:

- 1 and ½ cups cauliflower rice 2 cups coconut milk

- 3 tablespoons stevia

- 2 tablespoons ghee, melted

- 4 plums, pitted and roughly chopped

Directions:

1. In a bowl, mix all the ingredients, toss, divide into ramekins, put them in the air fryer, and cook at 340 degrees F for 25 minutes. Cool down and serve.

Nutrition: calories 221, fat 4, fiber 1, carbs 3, protein 3

Peanuts Almond Biscuits

Prep time: 20 minutes

Cooking time: 35 minutes

Servings: 6

Ingredients:

- 4 oz peanuts, chopped

- 2 tablespoons peanut butter

- ½ teaspoon apple cider vinegar

- 1 egg, beaten

- 6 oz almond flour

- ¼ cup of coconut milk

- 2 teaspoons Erythritol

- 1 teaspoon vanilla extract

- Cooking spray

Directions:

1.   In the bowl mix up peanut butter, apple cider vinegar, egg, almond flour, coconut milk, Erythritol, and

vanilla extract. When the mixture is homogenous, add peanuts and knead the smooth dough. Then spray the cooking mold with cooking spray and place the dough inside. Preheat the air fryer to 350F. Put the mold with biscuits in the air fryer and cook it for 25 minutes. Then slice the cooked biscuits into pieces and return back in the air fryer. Cook them for 10 minutes more. Cool the cooked biscuits completely.

Nutrition: calories 334, fat 29.1, fiber 5.2, carbs 10.8, protein 13.4

Walnuts and Almonds Granola

Preparation time: 4 minutes

Cooking time: 8 minutes

Servings: 6

Ingredients:

- cup avocado peeled, pitted and cubed

- ½ cup coconut flakes

- tablespoons ghee, melted

- ¼ cup walnuts, chopped

- ¼ cup almonds, chopped 2 tablespoons stevia

Directions:

1. In a pan that fits your air fryer, mix all the ingredients, toss, put the pan in the fryer and cook at 320 degrees F for 8 minutes. Divide into bowls and serve right away.

Nutrition: calories 170, fat 3, fiber 2, carbs 4, protein 3

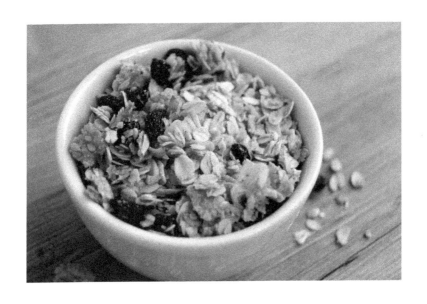

Cinnamon and Butter Pancakes

Prep time: 10 minutes

Cooking time: 12 minutes

Servings: 2

Ingredients:

- 1 teaspoon ground cinnamon
- 2 teaspoons butter, softened
- 1 teaspoon baking powder
- ½ teaspoon lemon juice
- ½ teaspoon vanilla extract
- ¼ cup heavy cream
- 4 tablespoons almond flour
- 2 teaspoons Erythritol

Directions:

1.   Preheat the air fryer to 325F. Take 2 small cake mold and line them with baking paper. After this, in the mixing bowl mix up ground cinnamon, butter, baking powder, lemon juice, vanilla extract, heavy cream,

almond flour, and Erythritol. Stir the mixture until it is smooth. Then pour the mixture in the prepared cake molds. Put the first cake mold in the air fryer and cook the pancake for 6 minutes. Then check if the pancake is cooked (it should have light brown color) and remove it from the air fryer. Repeat the same steps with the second pancake. It is recommended to serve the pancakes warm or hot.

Nutrition: calories 414, fat 37.4, fiber 6.7, carbs 14.7, protein 12.4

Hazelnut Vinegar Cookies

Prep time: 25 minutes

Cooking time: 11 minutes

Servings: 6

Ingredients:

- 1 tablespoon flaxseeds
- ¼ cup flax meal
- ½ cup coconut flour
- ½ teaspoon baking powder
- 1 oz hazelnuts, chopped
- 1 teaspoon apple cider vinegar
- 3 tablespoons coconut cream
- 1 tablespoon butter, softened
- 3 teaspoons Splenda
- Cooking spray

Directions:

1.   Put the flax meal in the bowl. Add flax seeds, coconut flour, baking powder, apple cider vinegar, and Splenda. Stir the mixture gently with the help of the fork and add butter, coconut cream, hazelnuts, and knead the non-sticky dough. If the dough is not sticky enough, add more coconut cream. Make the big ball from the dough and put it in the freezer for 10- 15 minutes. After this, preheat the air fryer to 365F. Make the small balls (cookies) from the flax meal dough and press them gently. Spray the air fryer basket with cooking spray from inside. Arrange the cookies in the air fryer basket in one layer (cook 3-4 cookies per one time) and cook them for 11 minutes. Then transfer the cooked cookies on the plate and cool them completely. Repeat the same steps with remaining uncooked cookies. Store the cookies in the glass jar with the closed lid.

Nutrition: calories 147, fat 10.3, fiber 6.3, carbs 11.1, protein 4.1

Sage Cream

Preparation time: 5 minutes

Cooking time: 30 minutes

Servings: 4

Ingredients:

- 7 cups red currants 1 cup swerve

- 1 cup water

- 6 sage leaves

Directions:

1. In a pan that fits your air fryer, mix all the ingredients, toss, put the pan in the fryer and cook at 330 degrees F for 30 minutes. Discard sage leaves, divide into cups and serve cold.

Nutrition: calories 171, fat 4, fiber 2, carbs 3, protein 6

Peanut Butter Cookies

Prep time: 30 minutes

Cooking time: 20 minutes

Servings: 4

Ingredients:

- ½ cup almond flour

- 2 tablespoons butter, softened

- 1 tablespoon Splenda

- ¼ teaspoon vanilla extract

- 4 teaspoons peanut butter

- 1 teaspoon Erythritol

- Cooking spray

Directions:

1. Make the cookies: put the almond flour and butter in the bowl. Add Splenda and vanilla extract and knead the non-sticky dough. Then cut dough on 8 pieces. Make the balls and press them to get the flat cookies. Preheat the air fryer to 365F. Spray the air fryer basket with

cooking spray and put the cookies in the air fryer in one layer – make 4 flat cookies per one time). Cook them for 10 minutes. Repeat the same steps with remaining cookies. Cool the cooked flat cookies completely. Meanwhile, mix up Erythritol and peanut butter. Then spread 4 flat cookies with peanut butter mixture and cover them with remaining cookies.

Nutrition: calories 118, fat 10.2, fiber 0.7, carbs 4.8, protein 2.1

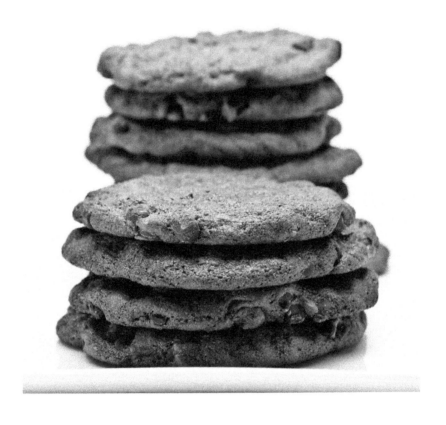

Currant Cream Ramekins

Preparation time: 5 minutes

Cooking time: 20 minutes

Servings: 6

Ingredients:

- 1 cup red currants, blended

- 1 cup black currants, blended 3 tablespoons stevia

- cup coconut cream

Directions:

1. In a bowl, combine all the ingredients and stir well. Divide into ramekins, put them in the fryer and cook at 340 degrees F for 20 minutes. Serve the pudding cold.

Nutrition: calories 200, fat 4, fiber 2, carbs 4, protein 6

Cilantro Cod Mi x

Preparation time: 5 minutes

Cooking time: 15 minutes

Servings: 4

Ingredients:

• 1 cup cherry tomatoes, halved Salt and black pepper to the taste 2 tablespoons olive oil

• 4 cod fillets, skinless and boneless 2 tablespoons cilantro, chopped

Directions:

1. In a baking dish that fits your air fryer, mix all the ingredients, toss gently, introduce in your air fryer and cook at 370 degrees F for 15 minutes.

2. Divide everything between plates and serve right away.

Nutrition: calories 248, fat 11, fiber 2, carbs 5, protein 11

Cayenne Salmon

Prep time: 10 minutes

Cooking time: 9 minutes

Servings: 3

Ingredients:

- 1-pound salmon

- 1 tablespoon Erythritol

- 1 tablespoon coconut oil, melted

- ½ teaspoon cayenne pepper

- 1 teaspoon water

- ¼ teaspoon ground nutmeg

Directions:

1. In the small bowl mix up Erythritol and water. Then rub the salmon with ground nutmeg and cayenne pepper. After this, brush the fish with Erythritol liquid and sprinkle with melted coconut oil. Put the salmon on the foil. Preheat the air fryer to 385F. Transfer the foil with salmon in the air fryer basket and cook for 9 minutes.

Nutrition: calories 241, fat 14, fiber 0.1, carbs 5.3, protein 29.4

Lemon and Oregano Tilapia Mix

Preparation time: 5 minutes

Cooking time: 20 minutes

Servings: 4

Ingredients:

•   4 tilapia fillets, boneless and halved Salt and black pepper to the taste

•   1 cup roasted peppers, chopped

•   ¼ cup keto tomato sauce 1 cup tomatoes, cubed

•   1 tablespoon lemon juice 2 tablespoons olive oil

•   1 teaspoon garlic powder 1 teaspoon oregano, dried

Directions:

1.   In a baking dish that fits your air fryer, mix the fish with all the other ingredients, toss, introduce in your air fryer and cook at 380 degrees F for 20 minutes. Divide into bowls and serve.

Nutrition: calories 250, fat 9, fiber 2, carbs 5, protein 14

Butter Lobster

Prep time: 10 minutes

Cooking time: 6 minutes

Servings: 4

Ingredients:

- 4 lobster tails, peeled

- 4 teaspoons almond butter

- ½ teaspoon salt

- ½ teaspoon dried thyme

- 1 tablespoon avocado oil

Directions:

1.   Make the cut on the back of every lobster tail and sprinkle them with dried thyme and salt. After this, sprinkle the lobster tails with avocado oil.

2.   Preheat the air fryer to 380F. Place the lobster tails in the air fryer basket and cook them for 5 minutes. After this, gently spread the lobster tails with almond butter and cook for 1 minute more.

Nutrition: calories 183, fat 10, fiber 1.8, carbs 4.,3, protein 20.5

Lemony Mustard Shrimp

Preparation time: 5 minutes

Cooking time: 12 minutes

Servings: 4

Ingredients:

- and ½ pounds shrimp, peeled and deveined Zest of ½ lemon, grated

- Juice of ½ lemon

- A pinch of salt and black pepper 2 tablespoons mustard

- tablespoons olive oil

- 2 tablespoons parsley, chopped

Directions:

1. In a bowl, mix all the ingredients and toss well. Put the shrimp in your air fryer's basket and reserve the lemon vinaigrette. Cook at 350 degrees F for 12 minutes, flipping the shrimp halfway, divide between plates and serve with reserved vinaigrette drizzled on top.

Nutrition: calories 202, fat 8, fiber 2, carbs 5, protein 14

Turmeric Fish Fingers

Prep time: 15 minutes

Cooking time: 9 minutes

Servings: 4

Ingredients:

- 1-pound cod fillet

- ½ cup almond flour

- 2 eggs, beaten

- ½ teaspoon ground turmeric

- 1 tablespoon flax meal

- 1 teaspoon salt

- 1 teaspoon avocado oil

Directions:

1.   Slice the cod fillets into the strips (fingers). In the mixing bowl, mix up eggs, ground turmeric, and salt. Stir the liquid until salt is dissolved. Then in the separated bowl mix up almond flour and flax meal. Dip the cod fingers in the egg mixture and coat in the almond flour

mixture. Preheat the air fryer to 400F. Place the fish fingers in the air fryer basket in one layer and sprinkle with avocado oil. Cook the fish fingers for 4 minutes.

2.   Then flip them on another side and cook for 5 minutes more or until the fish fingers are golden brown.

Nutrition: calories 153, fat 5.8, fiber 1, carbs 1.7, protein 24.2

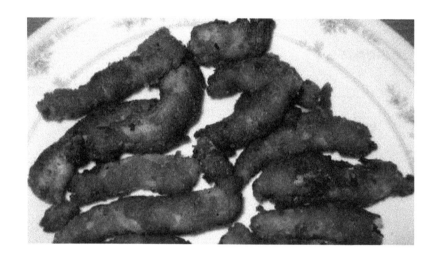

Parsley Shrimp

Preparation time: 5 minutes

Cooking time: 12 minutes

Servings: 4

Ingredients:

• pound shrimp, peeled and deveined 1 teaspoon cumin, ground

• tablespoons parsley, chopped 2 tablespoons olive oil

• A pinch of salt and black pepper 4 garlic cloves, minced

• 1 tablespoon lime juice

Directions:

1. In a pan that fits your air fryer, mix all the ingredients, toss, put the pan in your air fryer and cook at 370 degrees F and cook for 12 minutes, shaking the fryer halfway. Divide into bowls and serve.

Nutrition: calories 220, fat 11, fiber 2, carbs 5, protein 12

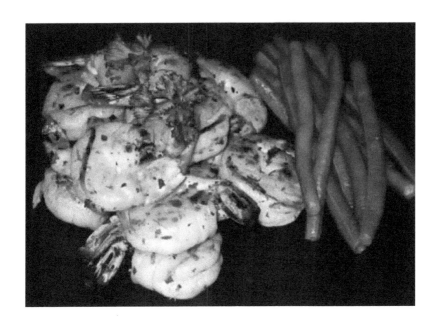

Herbed Salmon

Prep time: 10 minutes

Cooking time: 15 minutes

Servings: 4

Ingredients:

- ½ teaspoon dried rosemary
- ½ teaspoon dried thyme
- ½ teaspoon dried basil
- ½ teaspoon ground coriander
- ½ teaspoon ground cumin
- ½ teaspoon ground paprika
- ½ teaspoon salt
- 1-pound salmon
- 1 tablespoon olive oil

Directions:

1.   In the bowl mix up spices: dried rosemary, thyme, basil, coriander, cumin, paprika, and salt. After this,

gently rub the salmon with the spice mixture and sprinkle with olive oil. Preheat the air fryer to 375F. Line the air fryer with baking paper and put the prepared salmon inside. Cook the fish for 15 minutes or until you get the light crunchy crust.

Nutrition: calories 183, fat 10.6, fiber 0.2, carbs 0.4, protein 22.1

Ghee Shrimp and Green Beans

Preparation time: 5 minutes

Cooking time: 15 minutes

Servings: 4

Ingredients:

• pound shrimp, peeled and deveined A pinch of salt and black pepper

• ½ pound green beans, trimmed and halved Juice of 1 lime

• tablespoons cilantro, chopped

• ¼ cup ghee, melted

Directions:

1. In a pan that fits your air fryer, mix all the ingredients, toss, introduce in the fryer and cook at 360 degrees F for 15 minutes shaking the fryer halfway. Divide into bowls and serve.

Nutrition: calories 222, fat 8, fiber 3, carbs 5, protein 10

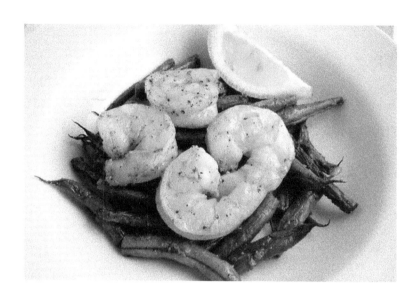

Basil Scallops

Prep time: 15 minutes

Cooking time: 6 minutes

Servings: 4

Ingredients:

- 12 oz scallops

- 1 tablespoon dried basil

- ½ teaspoon salt

- 1 tablespoon coconut oil, melted

Directions:

1. Mix up salt, coconut oil, and dried basil. Brush the scallops with basil mixture and leave for 5 minutes to marinate. Meanwhile, preheat the air fryer to 400F. Put the marinated scallops in the air fryer and sprinkle them with remaining coconut oil and basil mixture. Cook the scallops for 4 minutes. Then flip them on another side and cook for 2 minutes more.

Nutrition: calories 104, fat 4.1, fiber 0, carbs 2, protein 14.3

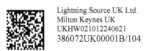

Lightning Source UK Ltd.
Milton Keynes UK
UKHW021012240621
386072UK00001B/104

9 781803 175713